QUESTION GOD

THE ANATOMY
OF AN
ASKING CHRISTIAN

By
Ralph Moore, M.D.

TEACH Services, Inc.
Brushton, New York

2008 09 10 11 12 · 5 4 3 2 1

Copyright © 2008 TEACH Services, Inc.
ISBN-13: 978-1-57258-509-6
ISBN-10: 1-57258-509-9
Library of Congress Control Number: 2007940660

Published by

TEACH Services, Inc.
www.TEACHServices.com

CONTENTS

INTRODUCTION

That I might more diligently seek the lord and hopefully come upon the evidences of His intended manner of approach to me, and the provisions He has made for my approach to Him, has been my prayer.

In this presentation I have expressed my own thoughts along with many statements from the inspired writings and from science and submit them to you for your own wonderment.

The first six chapters list some very remarkable claims taken from the Bible and from the Spirit of Prophecy that are almost beyond belief, and therefore must either be denied or must be accepted by faith alone.

Of course faith has its place but let us not miss the joys of reality. So the last eleven chapters list the facts and figures taken from proven and accepted scientific facts of physics, chemistry, anatomy, physiology and other phenomena of nature which verify the truth of these remarkable and outstanding statements of inspiration.

—Ralph B. Moore, M.D.

CHAPTER ONE

My Bible says that God made man in His own image. (Genesis 1:26) Did God run a risk? No! A risk is a situation in which there can be various and even unknown consequences. Sin and rebellion was no surprise to the Father and His dear Son. "The plan of redemption was not an afterthought... From the beginning God and Christ knew of the apostasy of Satan and the fall of man...God did not ordain that sin should exist, but He foresaw its existence and made provision for the terrible emergency."[1] This universal threat of sin and rebellion that would come into existence as a result of Lucifer's marvelous intellect and unlimited freedom, would require a universal remedy.

All this was "brooded in the mind of the Infinite, but kept in silence through times eternal."[2] "Our little world was to become the lesson book of the universe."[3] We are to sing a song to the universe: *"Redeemed! How I love to proclaim it! Redeemed by the blood of the Lamb; Redeemed through His infinite mercy, His child and forever I am."* (Fanny J. Crosby)

We know that, "the sufferings of Christ did not begin nor end with His manifestation in humanity, for the cross was but a faint revelation to our dull senses, of the pain, that from its very inception, sin has brought to the heart of God."[4]

No, the creation of Lucifer and of man did not create a risk. God does not run risks! Lucifer's jealousy and Adam's fall were foreknown and Christ's redemptive act was prearranged.

For Christ, however, there <u>was</u> an element of risk involved; an experiential risk. When Christ took upon

1   *Desire of Ages*, 22.
2   *Education*, 126.
3   *Desire of Ages*, 19.
4   *Education*, 263.

Himself the nature and weakness of fallen humanity, He had to surrender His foreknowledge of success in His great conflict with Satan, depending totally on the Father for strength and wisdom in response to the terrible onslaughts of Satan. "As a <u>man</u> He supplicated the throne till his body was charged with the heavenly current."[5] "Jesus had no advantage that we do not have. To Jesus, Who emptied Himself, was given the Holy Spirit without measure. So it may be with us."[6] As a man He must meet the most severe temptations of Satan without knowing that He would live through the ordeal without sinning. "He could have sinned. He could have fallen."[7]

"Satan wrung the heart of Jesus. On the cross the Savior could not see through the portals of the tomb. Hope did not present to Him, His coming forth from the grave a conqueror or tell Him of the Father's acceptance of His sacrifice."[8] In the darkness that surrounded Him, He cried, "My God! My God! Why has thou forsaken Me?" (Matthew 24:46) Not until the very last moment before death, "by faith He rested in Him whom it had ever been His joy to obey, and as in submission He committed Himself to God, the <u>sense of loss</u> of His Father's favor was withdrawn...and He cried, "It is finished. Father into Thy hands I commit My Spirit."[9]

Praise God for His infinite love and foresight. God realized He must allow the misery of sin because of the worthlessness of forced obedience. As Soon as there was sin, there was a Saviour. As soon as there was fear, there was a Father. As soon as there was misery, there was mercy. As soon as there was death, there was a Deliverer.

---

5   *Education*, 80, 81.
6   *Sons and Daughters*, 31
7   *SDA Bible Commentary*, *Vol. 5*, 1128.
8   *Desire of Ages*, 753, 754.
9   Ibid., 756

God moves in a mysterious way
His wonders to perform;
He plants His foot-steps in the sea
And rides upon the storm.

Ye fearful saints, fresh courage take;
The clouds ye so much dread
Are big with mercy, and shall break
With blessing on your head.

His purposes will ripen fast,
Unfolding every hour;
The bud may have a bitter taste,
But sweet will be the flower.

Blind unbelief is sure to err,
And scan His work in vain;
God is His own interpreter,
And He will make it plain.

Willliam Cowper, 1772

CHAPTER TWO

In the earliest of all beginnings, God had some exceedingly difficult choices to make. Would He create life or not? More importantly, what kind of life would he create? Would it be programmed like a computer to behave in certain ways? Would it be animal-like with instinctual behavior, but without conscience? Or would this highest level of creation be very similar to God Himself, with moral sensibilities and the freedom of each individual to choose his own destiny?

God's choice was made infinitely more difficult by His great wisdom and foreknowledge. He clearly saw that to allow free choice would lead to the horrors with which we now are all too familiar.

Foreseeing Lucifer's jealousies and deceptive activities, it seems that God saw the human race as the key to the remedy and as though it could "...could come to the kingdom for such a time as this." It was as though God had said, "Sin is here. Now let Us **HURRY** and finish this part of the plan with the **SPECIAL CREATION!**"

HURRY?? YES! "The Father consulted the Son in regard to **AT ONCE** carry out Their plan to make man...!"[10]

SPECIAL CREATION?? YES!! God said, "Let Us make man in Our image and after our likeness."[11] (Genesis 1:26) This was something new and different. Evidently previous creations had not been on this order. "Human beings were a new and distinct order," in that they were in the very image of God.[12]

We are instructed that, "We need to consider both the **NATURE** of man and the **PURPOSE**, of God in creating him."[13]

---

10 The Story of Redemption, 19
11 "SDA Bible Commentary, Vol. 1, 1081
12 Ibid.
13 Education, 713

The **NATURE** of man, "...a new and distinct order," in the "...very image of God," and of this new creation, "...except by his own choice, there was to be no limit to the possibilities of his development."[14] The mind of man was to be, "...brought in touch with the unseen mighty Intelligence; brought into communion with the mind of God, the finite with the Infinite...The effect of which is beyond estimate! "[15] This is the mystery of Godliness... that Christ should present His children to the Father to have conferred upon them an honor **EXCEEDING THAT CONFERRED UPON THE ANGELS**!!! This is the marvel of the heavenly universe."[16]

The **PURPOSE** was two fold:

(1) "For fellowship with God" ; "For companionship with Him,"[17]

(2) "After a time of test and trial...it was God's purpose to repopulate heaven with the human family."[18]

Think of it friends. We were created for a heritage like you've never dreamed of, but we stumbled and fell, and heaven has been a lonesome place ever since. But never-the-less, I thank God that He did not choose to create me as the animals or as robots, but that I stand free in the universe to make my own choices with no hidden buttons some higher power can push to make my decisions for me.

Once God made the decision to start creating things, it would not be possible for Him to remove even Lucifer from His creation plan, for if God with His foreknowledge were to eliminate before their creation, all beings who would choose against Him, would free choice be real? No. It would be a sham.

14 Ibid., 125
15 Ibid., 14
16 *Sons and Daughters*, 22; *Desire of Ages*, 21
17 *Education* 124; *Medical Ministry*, 48
18 *SDA Bible Commentary*, Vol. 1, 1082

An interesting sidelight here: [very debatable and most unreliable in this case]. There is a law in the study of probabilities that says in effect, that anything that can happen, if you wait long enough, it will happen. In the computations of integral calculus, if a situation can be expressed and integrated between zero and infinity, the possibility and the probability that it can happen, can be expressed. The physical and mathematical intricacies of zero versus infinity [eternity] are most challenging! How long Lucifer existed before evil was found in him, we do not know, but can it be seen that if sin is made possible, it must be considered inevitable or perhaps even necessary in order that it may be condemned without prejudice, ie permitted in order to be witnessed and witnessed in order to be judged and judged in order to be condemned and condemned in order to be destroyed. Arbitrary condemnation without a trial is considered as universally unfair. Since arbitrary condemnation is unfair, sin must be possible to be condemned. Integral Calculus (calculated integration) is no substitute for foreknowledge, but it surely can raise a host of questions!

The only other time God ever made anything like man was when He created Lucifer, for we are told, God created him... "as near as possible like Himself."[19] Now the human race being in that same order, Lucifer saw as a challenge to his position and he became jealous of Christ for not including him in the council regarding the creation of man.[20] Remember, Lucifer had a throne of his own radiant with light,[21] but now to this new creation (man), was eventually to be given the very highest privilege of "Sitting with Me [Christ] in My throne, even as I am set down with My Father in His throne." (Revelation 3:21) (See comment: *The Great Controversy*, 484)

God's plan for man was temporarily interrupted by Satan in the Garden of Eden; interrupted long enough to prove a point; a point that he is destined to become eminently prepared to prove: that God must annihilate

---

19 *SDA Bible Commentary*, Vol. 4, 1163
20 *The Story of Redemption*, 13, 14
21 *SDA Bible Commentary*, Vol. 7, 973

sin; that He will have a perfect right to do so, and that He has a people prepared to be His necessary and sufficient exhibit and proof of His need and right to do so.

This fallen and sinful race, through a love relationship, developed along a mutually thorny pathway with their Creator, is to become the means to perfectly justify the permanent and complete annihilation of sin from the universe. This relationship becomes so intimate that both the Creator and His created ones request that it never be altered; "Divinity and humanity combined in them."[22] "Mystically and eternally one."[23] What love! What infinite love! "Wonder Oh heavens and be astonished Oh earth."

Considering God's great love for this fallen human race, don't you know how very much He yearns to communicate that love to us? But He knows that He dares not be "pushy" in that endeavor. God desires very much to commune with us, His wayward children, but He does not force His presence upon us. That is not the way of love. But God is still God, oh precious thought. "Like the stars in the vast circuit of their appointed path, God's purposes know no haste and no delay."[24]

---

22 *SDA Bible Commentary*, Vol. 5, 1082
23 *Testimonies to Ministers*, 519; *Desire of Ages*, 25.
24 *Desire of Ages*, 32

CHAPTER THREE

If "God *SO* loved us, and with His infinite wisdom was capable of creating us, He certainly did not forget to install in us a very complete and effective system to accomplish His great desire; "...that we not only touch the hem of His garment, but walk with Him in <u>constant communion</u>."[25] Did he actually install such a system? "<u>Examine yourselves, prove your own selves</u>, how that <u>Christ is IN you</u>." (2 Corinthians 13:5) "Know ye not that your body is the temple of the Holy Ghost, which is <u>in you</u>, which ye have of God? (2 Corinthian 6:19) "The Lord Jesus loves His people, and when they put their trust wholly in Him, He will <u>live through</u> them, giving them the inspiration of His sanctifying Spirit, imparting to them a <u>vital transfusion</u> of Himself..."[26] "The love which Christ diffuses through the whole being is a <u>vitalizing power</u>... Every part...the brain, the heart, the nerves...<u>it touches</u>."[27] Is it necessary to ask, "Did God actually install a communication system in us?" "Oh Father," we pray, "Do not leave us without Your answer. Is there not more that we may know? May we, in some manner, draw nearer to You,—still nearer?"

Nearer, still nearer, close to Thy heart,
Draw me my Saviour, so precious Thou art;
Fold me, O fold me close to Thy breast,
Shelter me safe in that haven of rest.

C.H. Morris 1898

Is this communication arrangement literal or is it altogether figurative? Or is it here literal and there figurative? We are instructed to study and compare, "Here a

---

25   *The Ministry of Healing,* 85
26   *That I May Know Him,* 78
27   *The Ministry of Healing,* 115

little and there a little," but where does it all come to-
gether for the average person? What is the physiologic
and anatomic arrangement of our bodies in order to
fulfill our Father's desire to commune with us and we
with Him? May we look for such a provision? Is much
revealed? Again I read, "It is <u>no casual touch</u> with Christ
that we must have...but an <u>abiding in</u> him... This means
that you are to be <u>conscious</u> of an <u>abiding</u> Christ...Do not
stand outside of this experience...To <u>abide in Me</u> and <u>I in
you</u> is a possible thing to do."[28]

At this point many questions arise. How? Where?
Show Me! Are we on holy ground? Yes! Too Holy? Let us
look to inspired counsel. A few comments by inspiration
raises a word of caution.

"The <u>worldly</u> wise have attempted to explain on scientific principles, the influence of God upon the heart.
The least advance in this direction will lead the soul into
the mazes of skepticism."[29] "To the keenest intellect, that
Holy Being must ever be clothed in mystery."[30] "It is not
essential for us to define just <u>what</u> the Holy Spirit is...It
is plainly declared regarding the Holy Spirit, that "In His
work of guiding men into all truth, 'He shall not speak of
Himself.' The nature of the Holy Spirit is a mystery. Men
cannot explain it... Regarding such mysteries... silence is
golden."[31]

Again we ask, are we on holy ground? Yes! Forbidden
ground? Yes! For we have read, "Regarding such myster-
ies, silence is golden." <u>BUT</u> if we are <u>NOT</u> searching into
<u>WHAT</u> the Holy Spirit <u>IS</u>, are we not to learn His manner
and method of approach to us and the <u>PROVISIONS</u> God
has implanted within us for His access?

We read, "From the first dawn of reason, the human
mind should become intelligent in regard to its physical
structure, (Why?) for here Jehovah has given a <u>speci-
men</u> of Himself!"[32] "These grand principles are not to be

---

28   *In Heavenly Places*, 55
29   *Testimonies, Vol. 4*, 585
30   *SDA Bible Commentary, Vol. 7*, 904
31   *The Acts of Apostles*, 51, 52.
32   *Medical Ministry*, 221

thought too pure and too holy to be brought into the daily life. They are truths that reach to heaven and compass eternity, yet their vital influence is to be woven into human experience. They are to permeate all the great things and all the little things of life."[33] "Each person is to stand before God with an individual faith, an individual experience, knowing for himself that Christ is <u>formed within him</u>."[34] "With no limitation to the possibility of his development."[35] "Capable of communion with Him beyond estimate."[36] "It is our privilege to have a <u>living, abiding</u> Saviour, the Source of spiritual power, <u>implanted within</u> us."[37] "<u>Examine</u> yourselves, <u>prove</u> your ownselves...how that Christ is <u>in</u> you." (2 Corinthians, 13:5)

Certainly this is an invitation to seek a closer and more knowledgeable relationship with God. No! In this respect, we are not on forbidden ground, for, "When we approach God with a sincere desire and purpose to arrive at truth, we are <u>brought into touch</u> with the unseen, mighty Intelligence that is working **in** and **through** us ...The effect of such communion is beyond estimate."[38] "We can, we can...we can know the science of spiritual life."[39]

"When God's people put their trust in Him, depending wholly upon Him...He will live <u>through</u> them, giving them the impartation of His sanctifying Spirit, imparting to the soul a <u>vitalizing transfusion</u> of Himself, and <u>acting through their faculties</u>, causing them to choose His will... then they may say...Christ <u>liveth in</u> me."[40]

No, we are not on forbidden ground when we approach God with a sincere desire to know Him, for, "the work of faith in Christ is not the work of our nature but the work of God on human minds, <u>wrought in the very soul</u> by the Holy Spirit...With its justifying, sanctifying

33   *Faith I Live By*, 123
34   *Our High Calling*, 108
35   *Education*, 125
36   Ibid., 14
37   *God's Amazing Grace*, 119
38   *Education*, 14
39   *In Heavenly Places*, 43
40   *That I May Know Him*, 78

power, it is above what men call science. It is the science of eternal realities...so simple that a child can understand it and yet the most learned cannot explain it.[41] Can anyone explain a mother's love? No, but a child can experience it. "It is no casual touch with Christ...but an abiding in Him...This means that you are to be conscious of an abiding Christ...to abide in me and I in you is a possible thing to do. The invitation would not be given if you could not do this. Jesus is constantly drawing you with His Holy Spirit, working with your mind that you will abide with Christ."[42] "All we can bear of it [this kind of communion], we are invited to receive here."[43]

41   *In Heavenly Places*, 51
42   Ibid., 55
43   *Desire of Ages*, 331

CHAPTER FOUR

When Christ came to this earth, He came to make known to man the love of God. By precept and example, by parables, miracles and sermons, on the mountain side, in the valleys, by the sea, in the synagogue, by the wayside, in the city streets, in the workshop, and in the market place, He demonstrated not only the power of that love, but how to approach the Father by prayer, by praise and by applying the Word. How to commune with God, He demonstrated in human form. Jesus "communed with the Father till He was charged with the heavenly current then imparted that life to men. This perfect humanity we may possess for He used no power that we may not use."[44]

Do you now wonder what are the natural results that sincere suppliants may experience? "The sincere believer diffuses a vital energy which is penetrating and imparts a new moral power to souls for whom he labors. It is not the power of men, but of the Holy Spirit. Now we cannot give to others that which we ourselves do not possess. Unless the Holy Spirit uses us as agents through whom to communicate to the world the truth as it is in Jesus, we are...entirely useless."[45] "But he that believeth in Me, from within him shall <u>flow</u> rivers of living water." (John 7:38)

According to this we are permitted to be channels for the Holy Spirit! "The love of Christ as a healing, life giving <u>current</u> is to <u>flow through</u> your life."[46] Are we being lead to believe that the love of Christ is a <u>current</u> that <u>flows</u>?

Regarding this current of <u>virtue</u> do you recall the experience related in Luke 8:45, in which the woman with

44   *Education*, 80 and *Desire of Ages*, 664
45   *Thoughts from the Mount of Blessings*, 36
46   *The Ministry of Healing*, 156

the issue of blood for twelve years, said in her heart, "If I may but touch the hem of His garment, I shall be healed?" We usually emphasize the faith of the woman in this incident, but let us consider an equally interesting fact. The disciples were surprised that Jesus asked, "Who touched Me," because of the throng that surrounded Him, but Jesus said, "I perceive that <u>virtue</u> hath <u>gone out</u> of Me." Virtue <u>flowed out</u> of Christ. Again, in Luke 6:19 "The whole multitude sought to touch Him for there <u>went virtue out of Him</u> and healed them all." Commenting on the experience of the woman, Ellen White says, "He desires you not only to touch the hem of His garment, but to walk with Him in <u>constant communion</u>."[47] Oh! What an experience! Literally? Enoch! Elijah! Moses! Daniel! You? Me? "Higher than the highest human thought can reach is God's ideal for His children." You? Me?[48]

We reread those remarkable and inspiring words, "here (in the human race) Jehovah has given a <u>SPECIMEN OF HIMSELF</u>!!!"[49] Nothing was ever created before with such an elevated status! "Man was the CROWNING act of creation, made in the IMAGE OF GOD and designed to be HIS COUNTERPART."[50] "With no limitation to the possibility of his development."[51] "Capable of communion with Him beyond estimate."[52] This is the mystery of God-likeness. Do you know how inspiration defines the mystery of Godliness?

"This is the mystery of Godliness: That Christ should take human nature, and by a life of humiliation, elevate man in the scale of moral worth with God; that He should carry His adopted nature to the throne of God, and there present His children to His Father, to have conferred upon them an honor EXCEEDING that conferred upon the angels! This is the marvel of the heavenly universe."[53]

---

47 *Ministry of Healing*, 85
48 *Education*, 18
49 *Medical Ministry*, 221
50 *The Review and Herald*, 06/18/1885
51 *Education*, 125
52 *Education*, 14
53 *Sons and Daughters*, 22.

What really does it mean as we recall the prayer of Jesus: "That they [His people] may be one with Him as He is one with the Father." (John 17:21) and to "Sit with Me in My throne even as I am also set down with My Father in His throne." (Revelation 3:21) Truly as we meditate upon these words, we can only stand back and marvel concerning God's love and His yearning to take us back home and to shower us with a love that only Jesus Himself can express! Oh Friend, let the tears of joy and praise flow freely from your love starved soul for the wonderful love of Jesus.

In Joyful high and holy lays,
My soul her grateful voice would raise;
But who can sing the worthy praise
Of the wonderful love of Jesus?

A joy by day, a peace by night,
In storm a calm, in darkness light,
In pain a balm, in weakness might,
Is the wonderful love of Jesus.

—E. D. Mund

We recognize that, "The sincere believer" who "diffuses a vital energy which is penetrating and imparts a new moral power to souls for whom he labors,"[54] represents an unusual experience and is an unusual believer, and is enjoying a rather advanced stage of sanctification and communion with his Creator. But we must admit, there really was an Enoch, an Elijah, A Moses, A Daniel and many others. The fact **is** there **is** the possibility for this miraculous experience to exist in human flesh.

These men of old that we have listed, were leaders among God's people, and where there was one leader, there were by comparison many followers who were sincere and will be in God's kingdom, so we may assume that this close communion is not uncommon among sincere believers.

---

54 *Thoughts from the Mount of Blessings*, 36

CHAPTER FIVE

It is not the purpose of this discourse to suggest that we travel around trying to get a photo of, or otherwise "catch" virtue flowing into or out of a Christian, for this cannot be. Even the mention of it seems sacrilegious. The work and activity of the Holy Spirit must ever remain a mystery. That is a most sacred territory, and concerning it, "silence is golden."

The theme of our study is not to analyze the Holy Spirit; not even to analyze His work, but to analyze ourselves,—anatomically. All we ask; is there a PROVISION or PROVISIONS that God has installed within the human machine that lends itself to the access of the influence of the Holy Spirit?

What does Philippians 2:5 say to us? "Let this mind be in you which was also in Christ Jesus." What does it mean in John 14: 17-21?..."but ye know Him; for He <u>dwelleth in you</u> and shall be <u>in you</u>...at that day ye shall know that I am in the Father, and ye in Me and <u>I in you</u>...and I will <u>MANIFEST</u> Myself to you."

Do you know just what we are asking? In all sincerity and reverence, we are asking, how does the Holy Spirit manifest Himself to us? Truly we believe that He does dwell in us. Can we know more? We have many pet phrases that we glibly voice to show our "great understanding" of a process we call, "coming to Jesus," but of which we know very little. We sing the song, *"Let Jesus Come Into Your Heart"* or we say "Just surrender your will to Jesus," "Reach out and take His hand," "Fall on the Rock and be broken", "Get a new life from above," "Just open your heart's door," "Behold the Lamb," Look to Jesus," "Give up on self," *"Trust and Obey, there's not other way,"* "Take Jesus at His Word," etc. Are we always learning new phrases and never coming to a knowledge of truth?

Jesus had this problem with the people too, so He taught them in parables. In Matthew 13:10,11,13 the disciples asked Jesus, "Why speakest Thou to them in parables?" Jesus answered, "Because it is given to <u>you</u> to <u>know</u> the mysteries of the kingdom of heaven, but to them it is not given...because they seeing, see not, neither do they understand," and Mark 4:33, "With many such parables spake He the Word as they were <u>able</u> hear it." Truth must be carefully presented. "Don't cut off the ears of the hearers who are not ready."[55]

The prophets of old prophesied of Jesus, "I will open my mouth in parables. I will utter things that have been kept secret from the foundation of the world." (Psalms 78: 1–7) When we hear it do we try to understand it, or do we say, "Nobody really understands it so why should I expect to understand it?" Do we desire to hear and understand it?

The time was ripe. Jesus was on earth. What could be the secret that they needed to begin to understand? Was it the PROVISION for the indwelling? The new covenant? The process of the communion of the Holy Spirit? Their new and unlimited access to the Holy Spirit that they were about to enjoy at Pentecost? The sanctifying process of the Holy Spirit that Jesus yearned to reveal to them? This was a hard thing for the disciples to understand. Is it a hard thing for us to understand?

"Even the mystery that hath been hid from ages and from generations, but now is <u>MADE MANIFEST</u> to His saints: to whom God would make known what is the riches of the glory of this mystery, which is <u>CHRIST IN YOU</u>, the hope of glory." (Colossians 1:26)—Oh—Read that last sentence again, one phrase at a time, slowly.

Jesus fulfilled this long awaited promise of the new covenant of Jeremiah; "I will put My law in their <u>inward parts</u> and write it in their hearts." (Jeremiah 31: 31–33) "Behold thou desirest truth in the <u>inward parts</u>. In the <u>hidden part</u> thou shalt make me to know wisdom." (Psalms 51:6)

Where are the hidden parts where we know and experience wisdom? Could it be our minds, our brains, our nervous system? Where else could it be?

The ancients had <u>inward parts</u> too. What is different for us? The ancients had access to salvation too. What is the difference for us? No difference, except that we are on this side of the cross and merely more able to observe the technicalities of the outworking of the plan of salvation.

Wouldn't you like to look into the electron microscope of today and see the processes of salvation; the pathways of the Holy Spirit? No! Not <u>virtue flowing</u>, but the <u>PROVISIONS</u> of our nervous system which the Holy Spirit uses in fulfilling our spiritual needs. Yes, the work of the Holy Spirit has always been and always will be, by <u>FAITH</u> and <u>FAITH ALONE</u>. But let us keep the equipment He uses in good shape for His use. What better way to keep in good condition than to understand its workings? "From the first dawn of reason, the human mind should become intelligent in regard to its physical structure. Why? For here Jehovah has given a <u>SPECIMEN</u> of <u>HIMSELF</u>."[56] "Man, the <u>CROWNING ACT</u> of creation...<u>HIS COUNTERPART!</u>"[57] "God would have His servants become acquainted with the moral machinery of their minds."[58]

What does it profit us to look into the machinery of the mind? "He, {God] in mercy reveals the hidden defects, that they may look within and examine critically the complicated emotions and exercises of their own hearts and detect that which is wrong; thus they may modify their disposition."[59]

In studying the effects of the action of the Holy Spirit on the mind, we must recognize that there are other approaches to the mind made by pseudoscience, psychics and the occult. We are cautioned against speculating concerning the powers of the mind, so let us avoid all curiosity approaches. So let us limit our study to the Bible and the inspired writings, the simple laws of physiology and

---

56 *Medical Ministry*, 221
57 *Review and Herald* 06/18/1895
58 *Testimonies, Vol. 4*, 85
59 *Testimonies, Vol. 4*, 85

the observable structures of our anatomy. With these safe limits, do we accept that there is a <u>living</u> relationship between God and His people? Yes, for when He was here on earth He sought every avenue to portray and bind up this personal relationship by His own precepts and example.

The nominal Christian does not believe that Christ has really touched him in a literal, physical sense. He glibly quotes, "I am crucified with CHRIST, nevertheless I live, yet not I, but Christ liveth in me." (Galatians 2:20) But to him spiritual life is not as real as physical life. He retreats into vagueness with a plea of reverence. A lot of intellectual ignorance, or maybe sinning, is hidden under the old aphorism of "thus far and no farther" of ancient script. (Job 38:11) He thinks of spiritual life as if it were contained in a bucket up in the sky and an angel tips the bucket every now and then and spills a little sincere milk of the word on a poor starving Christian when it sees him pale and spiritually short of breath. Spiritual life is not a myth, neither is it as much of a mystery as we consign it to be. We must understand the difference between myth and mystery. Myth is usually hearsay and most frequently false.

Mystery is a fact that either cannot or has not been explained. The margin of the lips of mystery are clean; not so with a myth. Paul gave an example of a mystery. "Behold I show you a mystery; we shall not all sleep, but we shall be changed." (1 Corinthians 15:51) How do you classify these texts: "Ye are the temple of the Living God: as God hath said, I will <u>dwell</u> in them and <u>walk in</u> them." (2 Corinthians 6:16) "Lord how is it that Thou wilt <u>MANI-FEST</u> Thyself into us... My Father and I...will come unto him and make Our <u>ABODE</u> with him." (John 14: 22,23)

Paul speaks more positively about it: "Know ye not that your <u>body is</u> the <u>temple</u> of the Holy Ghost, which <u>is in</u> you, which ye have of God." (1 Corinthians 6:19) "Examine yourselves, prove your own selves, know ye not your own selves how that Christ is in you, except ye be reprobates?" (2 Corinthians 13:5) "Ye are a holy temple of the Lord...for an <u>habitation of God.</u>" (Ephesians 2:21)

Oh, I say, surely this must impress you as being more than myth and more than figurative language, for the command is, "Be <u>filled</u> with the Spirit." "The continual cry of the heart is, 'more of Thee,' and ever the Spirit's answer, 'much more.'"[60] "All that human nature can bear, we may receive here."[61]

Surely, there will always be questions and mysteries, but the clouds of mystery do not descend until we have determined the most important truth that Jesus desired to impart to us, and that is, Christ is in the Christian. "The Holy Spirit is to be in us a DIVINE INDWELLER."[62] "To Jesus Who emptied Himself was given the Spirit without measure. So it may be with us."[63] "We must look for the sanctifying influence of the Holy Spirit, each in his own life."[64]

---

60 *God's Amazing Grace*, 213
61 *Desire of Ages*, 331
62 *Healthful Living*, 301
63 *Healthful Living*, 301
64 *God's Amazing Grace*, 219

CHAPTER SIX

We have thus far quoted many references that have pointed to the fact that Christians have a need to identify in some manner with their Creator and that God has manifested His yearning to fulfill that need of communion with Him. We have recognized the dangers of uncontrolled speculations and unauthorized approaches, but we have determined that a God Who loves us <u>so</u> much, yet Who must ever be clothed in mystery, is not going to let mystery stand in the way of our knowing Him, experiencing his presence and communing with him. '"For Christ does not deal with us in abstract theories, but in that which is essential...to enlarge our capacity to <u>know</u> God,...He speaks of those things that relate to the conduct of our life and that take hold of eternal realities."[65] Luther Warren was asked, "How is your faith?" his answer; "I have no faith, it is all reality."

I hope we are prepared to enter into the world of reality and to connect that which we have always known as reality with that which we have heretofore considered a mystery, but which in fact has itself always been reality. No, not how the Holy Spirit dwells in us, but how the nervous system has a marvelous PROVISION for the indwelling of the Holy Spirit and for responding to His presence, so that perhaps what previously has only been figurative, may burst upon you as a whole new reality. Let's call it THE NERVOUS SYSTEM OF THE CHRISTIAN. Oh yes, the nervous system of a Christian is remarkably different from that of a non-Christian,—literally, physically, structurally. "But," you say, "We are still dealing with statements that we are expected to accept by faith. When do we get down to those things that have mass and occupy space and that display physical evidence. Do we ever get away from having to take everything by faith?"

The answer to that is, and never will be otherwise, friend; "Christ must abide in us by FAITH...this in its <u>fullness</u> comes to us through <u>constant communion </u>with God...Christ and the Holy Spirit give us this <u>nerve pow-er</u>."[66] Read that again! This abiding, by a repetitious communion, develops a <u>fullness</u>! Incidently, right there on that point, have you never read that "Faith is a <u>Sub-stance</u>"...and that "it is <u>Evidence</u>?" (Hebrews 11:1) Let's begin to search through the <u>substance</u> of the nervous system, looking for the <u>evidence</u> that before the days of the electron microscope and a few other sensitive instru-ments, was "<u>Not seen</u>."

We need to understand how our brain functions and how it literally, in the flesh, can be reconstructed under the influence of the Holy Spirit. If, "Let this mind be in you which was also in Christ Jesus," (Philippians 2.5) is a possible thing to do, then you can say, "I live, yet not I, but Christ liveth in Me." (Galatians 2:20) These are not just promises but they are commands of the Most High.

"But," again you are asking, "How can I...Just wait now, remember the sheep and the goats? Sheep follow on to know the Lord, but goats—Butt? Now as you were about to say, "How can I, relatively speaking, compare my mind with the mind of God? Whatever has happened to that admonition and sense of humility?" We are not considering humility here, for as we have just said, these are not merely promises of accomplishment, but the com-mands of accomplishment by the Most High. "Ye shall be holy unto Me, for I the Lord *am* holy, and have severed you from other people, that ye should be Mine." (Leviti-cus 20:26) "What ever is to be done by His command may be accomplished in His strength. All His biddings are enablings."[67] Speaking of humility, most of our hu-mility as well as other excuses for not attaining to per-fection of character are merely efforts to get us off the "hook." Often we compare ourselves with another who seems to be having no problem in his Christian experi-

---

66   *Counsels on Health*, 593

67   *Christ's Object Lessons*, 333

ence and who is recognized as being a strong leader in the church. Just because we consider ourselves, relatively speaking, almost as good as someone else, or twice as good for that matter, is no evidence that God is grading us on the curve, or that He is using anyone else but Himself as the standard. Living up to God's standard or living up to the average Christian standard is two different ways of living, relatively speaking; and did you ever hear of being relatively saved? The command is, "Be ye therefore perfect, even as your Father which is in heaven is perfect." (Matthew 5:48) You will not be going around forgiving sins and creating new worlds as He can. No, of course not; but in that little cubicle where resides your personal developing character, by a provision and direction of a loving heavenly Father, there will be reborn a perfect reproduction, a mirror image of the character of Christ. How I would hate to think that with God himself accomplishing this, <u>in</u> and <u>for</u> us, we could expect or desire anything less than a perfect job!

"My, my, my, why did we have to take such a detailed, repetitious, and circuitous approach to this subject," you ask? Frankly, a lot of persuasive evidence under the guise of faith is sometimes necessary to persuade a skeptical soul that what he still would desire to remain as figurative phrases, is after all, factual commands, his past hopes and beliefs not withstanding.

Now that you have your answer and I'm "off the hook," let's proceed, using the care and detail that is needed when entering the arena where we had better start singing the song, *"Tread softly, tread softly, the Master is here."*

CHAPTER SEVEN

So now, <u>The Nervous System of the Christian</u>.

After a few brief statistics and a brief outline as a springboard to further stretch your considerations and develop your faith, let's embark on a little side trip into the nervous system. Perhaps a whole new and enjoyable area of reality will unfold before you as you observe how the promises of holy writ are fulfilled in scientific facts.

The usual explanation of the "new birth" experience is based entirely on one of the three postulates:

(1) That is it a myth, even though delivered in all sincerity by a religious enthusiast, and is accepted as just an earnest "sales pitch."

(2) That it is a hopeful supposition since some biblical prophecies did apparently have historical fulfillment.

(3) By faith alone it is accepted, although many biblical fulfillments do encourage and support that faith.

In this presentation we will review facts, figures and some rational and scientific conclusions that support the fact that the human agent is not merely trying to <u>improve his conduct</u> to meet God's approval, but that there is a built-in **PROVISION** that enables an anatomical <u>change</u> to be made to enable him to meet the mind of God.

The Central Nervous System (CNS) is made up of 10 to 12 billion cells, called neurons. Most neurons are visible only under a high powered electron microscope. They vary in length from a fraction of a millimeter to several feet. Three fourths of them are located in the gray matter (cortex) of the brain. That's the thin outer layer of the brain that is of such tremendous complexity and importance. Messages travel over these neurons by electrical impulses. No, not like the electron flow in a metal wire, but by "induced charges." These impulses (messages) travel at different speeds, varying from 2 miles per hour to 200 miles per hour. Just imagine, if you placed all of the neurons of the CNS side by side an inch apart, they would reach eight times around the world! Well maybe it would be easier to just count them, day and night and as fast as you can count. You couldn't do it. Not in your lifetime. No, for it would require more than six lifetimes!

The average person uses only between one and four percent of the available neurons. That's not surprising, for you see God originally intended to commune with us in a manner "beyond estimate"[68] but due to Adam's fall He had to put that idea on hold for a while.

"The relation that exists between the mind and the body is very intimate. Between the mind and the body there is a mysterious and wonderful relation. When one is affected the other sympathizes."[69] "The brain being the citadel of the being, wrong physical habits affect the brain."[70] and conversely the brain affects the body. "Therefore, keep the heart (mind) with all diligence, for out of it are the <u>issues</u> of <u>life</u>." (Proverbs 4:23)

Yes, the mind and the body were intended to act as a congenial whole, but in this old world of hurry and scurry, sometimes the <u>mind</u> finds the <u>body</u> is acting independently of it. For example, suppose I am walking down the street, thinking about getting to work on time, a "don't delay me attitude." I met Mr. King and I say with my mouth, (that's a part of my body):

My Body Action	My Thoughts
I say, "Good morning Mr. King"	It's not a good morning at all, and you certainly don't look like a King, dirty and all.
"How are you," I say	Oh please don't tell me that long sad tale of woe again.

---

68 *Education*, 14.
69 *Testimonies, Vol. 3*, 485
70 *Counsels to Parents, Teachers and Students*, 299

He asks me in turn, "How are you?	
"Fine," I say.	I'm not fine at all. In fact I don't feel so well.
I say, "Well, I'm glad, you surely are looking well this morning."	I'm not glad at all. In fact I never gave it a second thought. Actually you look kind'a sick,—dirty and pale. I wonder if he ever takes a bath.
So I put out my hand and say, How do you do?"	That silly old "how-dya'do"

I wonder who started it? Actually, I don't care how you do, or if you ever do anything at all. This shaking hands business is silly actually, germ transfer and all. Yes he still has those warts on his fingers. I hope they're not catching. They say they are of viral origin. Let go quick, man.

You smile, but often down in your heart (mind) you are thinking differently. Your face may be "putting on" a forced expression while your mind may be experiencing various attitudes of anxiety, remorse, hate, guilt, discontent, sorrow, envy, insecurity or fear. These mental attitudes can result in a real physical illness. Since the mind controls the body, these messages of unhappiness are carried to the organs of the body and their functions are impaired. "The condition of the mind affects the health to a far greater extent than many realize.[71]

---

71 *Ministry of Healing*, 241

CHAPTER EIGHT

The Holy Spirit picks up where you leave off! He will work with what He finds. There are a number of basic functions that He finds in your CNS. These functions may be highly developed in one direction or another, or in several directions. It is possible they have hardly been developed at all. The process is the same in any case. You resign, He designs. Precious Saviour...

Just when I need Him,
Jesus is near.
Just when I falter,
Just when I fear.
Ready to help me,
Ready to cheer.
Just when I need Him most.

Just when I need Him,
He is my all.
Answering when
Upon Him I call.
Tenderly watching,
Lest I should fall.
Just when I need Him most.
                    —William C. Poole 1897

Here we present a very simple outline of the CNS (Central Nervous System).

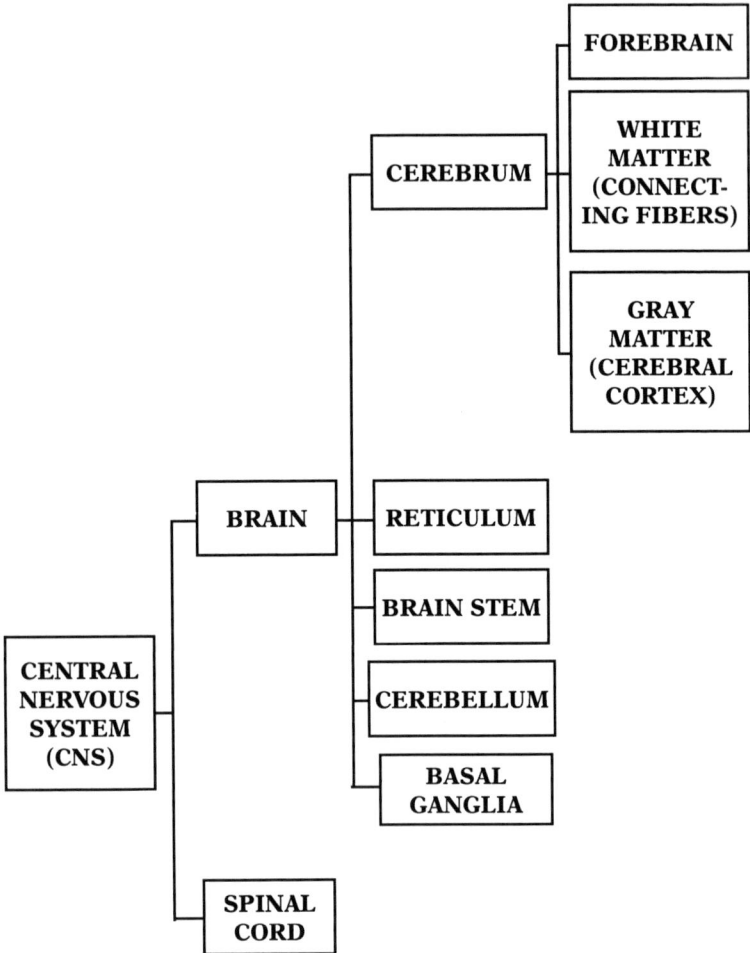

Now you would think from looking at this diagram of the CNS, that we would start at the top and work down in discussing it, but starting at the bottom and working up is much more rewarding. You'll see!

SPINAL CORD: Basic reflexes are based here. If you accidently put your finger on a hot stove, you automatically jerk it away. If you trip over something, you automatically thrust your arms forward. If something flies past your face, you automatically blink your eyes. These are <u>spinal</u> reflexes. There is not time for a conscious thought process to take place before damage might be inflicted. Our thoughtful Creator provided a short cut; the spinal reflex arc. A sensory nerve carries the hot finger message to the spinal cord. A short "reflex arc" connects to a motor nerve in the spine, which tells the arm muscle to retract the arm from the hot stove. Of course, a memo is sent to the brain to suspect all black stoves in the future, but the short cut "reflex arc" is just another way of showing God's concern for us. This is the most basic type of sensory message to motor response arrangement that exists in the body. It is present in all creatures; even at birth it is already present. The lowly earthworm coming up to an object, bumps into it, backs off, moves a little to the side, goes forward again, bumps again, moves aside again, goes forward and eventually goes around or over an obstruction. The lowly earthworm has only about twenty neurons in its nervous system!

BASAL GANGLIA: It is present in all creatures to a greater or lesser degree. It is the great generator of emotions and reactions; love, hate, fight, scream, kill, gross recognition of friend or foe situations, and all of the basic life support mechanisms.

CEREBELLUM: It really initiates nothing of itself, but rides herd on many things, such as making smooth, graceful movements of the body that otherwise would be floppy and jerky. It maintains muscle tone between movements such that they are not caught off guard. Bodily motion skills are honed to a fine degree.

BRAIN STEM: The basic control center for heart rate, respiration, blood pressure, digestion control, cough, sneeze, vomit, swallow (try to stop a swallow in mid-act!), automatic eye adjustments for focus, direction, accommodation to light, and much more.

RETICULUM: A very sensitive and important "immigration office" for incoming sensory messages, located at the top of the brain stem. Millions of impulses come and go from the higher centers of the brain and from the lower basic areas every second of your life, here to be sorted out. The higher control centers of the brain have pre-programmed the Reticulum to allow only a few of the highest priority messages through and have told the Reticulum to handle the great majority of messages as it has previously been instructed to do. For example, you move into a house right next to the railroad track and the passing train sounds as if it is coming right through the bedroom the first few nights, but your higher cerebral centers tell the Reticulum to ignore it, that it's unimportant. Very soon you hardly pay attention to it and it never awakens you at night anymore.

Your Reticulum can be programmed to prefer good or bad music, proper or junk foods. It can prioritize your interests on a graded scale of merit. It can remind you to pray and study your Bible. It will learn to forget if you deliberately neglect to follow the program you have previously taught it.

The Reticulum is the place good habits are formed. Or by neglect they are forgotten. This is the place bad habits are formed, and only by conscious effort can be broken. You, from the higher brain centers can program it.

Deliberate experiences will program it.
Random experiences will program it.
If you ask, the Holy Spirit will program it.
If you neglect, the devil will program it.

The Reticulum is a remarkable area, take care.
It is a dangerous area, beware.
"Choose ye this day,
Whom you will serve!" (Joshua 24:15)

CEREBRUM: That wonderful mass of **gray matter** and **white matter** that occupies the greater portion of the skull. The gray matter being the billions of neuron cell bodies and the white matter being the connecting fibers to all other parts of the CNS.

The gray matter is that thin gray outer layer of the cerebrum called Cerebral Cortex. We have mentioned that the Reticulum must be programmed. The Cortex is the originator of that Reticulum program. The white matter is that mass of connecting fibers to the rest of the CNS. The cortex is the most "conscious" area of the CNS. Many of it's areas if damaged will cause the person to become unconscious, while the lower CNS levels may carry on the basic functions of life support for days or years.

Mammals have certain mental capabilities over and above the lower creatures. Mammals are able to:

(1) **Store** tremendous amounts of information in the form of memory for use in later life. The horse, elephant, dog and baboon demonstrate this capability to various extents. In man this reaches its highest development. Man has the greatest brain size to body size ratio of all living organisms.

(2) **Think and Reason:** Thoughts and reasoning is largely a matter of memory juggling and logic. Also, it is the combining of previous experience with present incoming stimuli from the five senses. For example, while seeing and hearing a choir performance, these two senses are combined with previous memories of your own choir membership of many years past, allowing you to float through a very enjoyable mental side trip.

(3) **Communication:** Along with our memory and logic, we transmit by voice and written symbols, and receive by eye and ear.

(4) **Skills:** Though a major share of the motor function of
the body can be performed without the Cortex, one of
the distinguishing features of the human is its ability to
carry out extremely complex voluntary types of muscle
activity. It can perform the intricate task of talking,
writing, construction, playing a musical instrument,
all of which involves a high degree of control by the
Cerebral Cortex; then add the complexities of talent
and inherited predispositions!

Forebrain: (Of the Cerebrum) This is the "Master Control Room" where all conscious impulses can be observed
and where they can be called up and caused to pass in
review and made to give account of themselves. This is
the place of Judgment.

> What did I do?
>> What should I do?
>>> What will I do?
>>>> What should I have done?

Most of the principle decisions of daily life have previously been settled in the Forebrain and assigned to the
various lower habituated or semi-habituated areas of the
CNS, but here in the Forebrain is the area of judgement,
reason, concern, conscience, emotional review, discrimi-
nation, ethics, allegiance, responsibility, appreciation,
obligation, planning, rationalizing, imagination, inven-
tion and all of the problems and joys of life that must be
studied, re-evaluated, put on hold or acted upon. Truly
a strange and unique, over-ruling area, distinguishing
the desirable and undesirable as compared to the previously established standards; standards that were established here in the Forebrain at an earlier time. This is the
place that decides if the standards should be changed;
the center that determines for each individual, the ideals
by which he lives.

Up from the Basal Ganglia come POSITIVE emotions of:

Love
    Obligation
        Loyalty
           Courage
              Morality
                Hope
                  Ambition
                    Appreciation
                      Ethics

Up from the Basal Ganglia come NEGATIVE emotions of

Hate
    Defensiveness
        Revenge
           Fear
              Sorrow
                Selfishness
                  Guilt
                    Immorality
                    Remorse

All of these pouring into the Super Control Area to seek acceptance and demand action.

The Basal Ganglia Says	The Forebrain Says
Fight!	No, He's a Human being, a friend, an American.
Scream!	No, You're in Church.
Laugh!	No, You're at a Funeral.
Cry!	No, It's too embarrassing, you're a man.
Growl!	No, You're a Lady, not a dog.
Kill!	No, He's your brother, besides it's unlawful.
Escape!	No, Remain loyal to the cause.

THE FOREBRAIN

This is the Seat of Conscience
This is the Throne Room
This is the Citadel of the Soul
This is the Home of the Will
This is the Court of Final Appeal

Here Takes Place

The great Battle between Truth and Error
The Great War between Good and Evil
The GREAT CONTROVERSY BETWEEN
CHRIST AND SATAN

CHAPTER NINE

Does our loving Father want to meet with us, commune with us, speak with us, speak very personally with us; how do you suppose, from how far away. In old covenant times He said, *"Let them make Me a sanctuary, that I may DWELL AMONG* **them.**" (Exodus 25:8) Under the new covenant relationship, He desires to *DWELL IN* us. "God has prepared for Himself this <u>living habitation of the mind</u>. It is curiously wrought. A temple which the Lord Himself has fitted up for the <u>indwelling</u> of the Creator."[72]

Our Father talks about sealing us with His seal. Where do you suppose He will impress it? "And I saw another angel ascending from the East having the Seal of the Living God, and he cried...hurt not...till we have sealed the servants of our God in their forehead." (Revelation 7:2) Does Satan have a seal? Where does he seal his followers? "And he caused all...to receive a mark in the right hand or the forehead." (Revelation 13:16) What is just behind of the forehead where those seals are impressed? Yes, the <u>Forebrain</u>! That is really what is being sealed! Remember the Forebrain, the Citadel of the Soul, the Throne Room, the Seat of Conscience, the Home of the Will? The Seal of God is to be impressed on the Forebrain and programmed by it right on down to your toes! Just wait and See! "The <u>nerves of the brain</u> are the only medium through which heaven communicates with man and affects his innermost life. "[73]

Are we speaking in realities? Let us move forward, looking for more precious evidences.

---

72   *Desire of Ages*, 161
73   *Education*, 209

Precious Name
Oh, how sweet,
Hope of Earth
and Joy of Heaven!

CHAPTER TEN

Assuming that you have followed thus far, by a combination of faith and reality, will you allow your mind to stretch a little Farther? I want to comment on a still more profound aspect of the nervous system of the Christian - an aspect into the more intimate reality of the PROVISION available (but only with our consent) for the working of the Holy Spirit. I don't want to limit-- Oh No! Who would want to limit or dare to think of limiting the work of the Holy Spirit to a measurable or finite scale? "For there is no limit to the usefulness of one who putting self aside, makes room for the working of the Holy Spirit on his heart...to such ones...is given power for the attainment of measureless results...even in this life shall be seen the fulfillment of the promise of the future state![74]—But there are PROVISIONS that can be measured on finite scales!

At this stage in our study we must look further into the physical activity of neurons. Please enter into it with eager anticipation and understanding for the rewards are quite beyond description. "Oh, we can, we can...we can know the science of Spiritual life."[75] "There is a science of Christianity to be mastered—a science as much deeper, broader, higher, than any human science as the heavens are higher than the earth. The mind is to be disciplined, educated, trained; for we are to do service for God in ways that are not in harmony with inborn inclination... Our hearts must be educated to become steadfast in God. We are to form habits of thought that will enable us to resist temptation. By a life of holy endeavor and firm adherence to the right the children of God are to <u>seal</u> their destiny."[76]

---

74   *Desire of Ages*, 159, 160
75   *In Heavenly Places*, 43
76   Ibid., 26

Remember we said that the neurons are the building blocks of the nervous system. Though magnified a thousand times, it would still be smaller than a pin point, and though it may be bombarded with hundreds of impulses of information simultaneously, a neuron can process all that data and come out with the proper decision in less than a thousandth of a second.

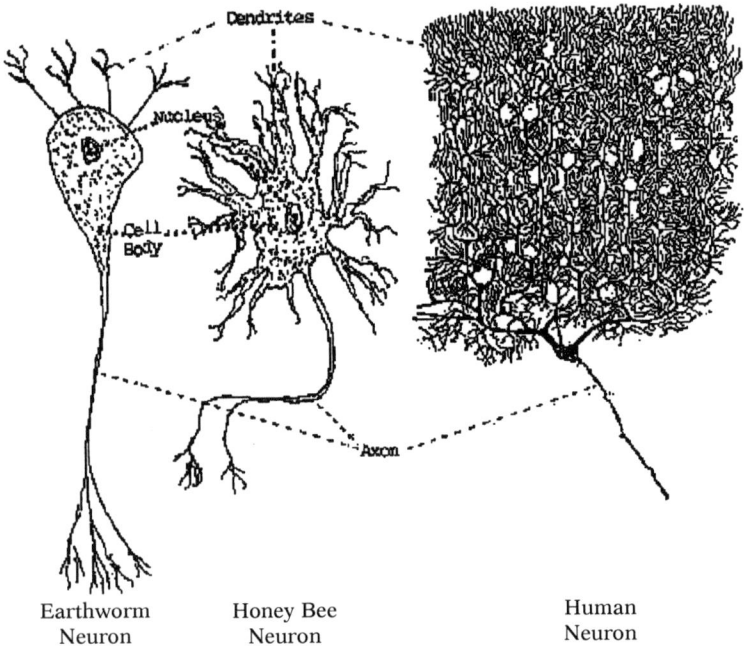

Dendrites
Nucleus
Cell Body
Axon

| Earthworm Neuron | Honey Bee Neuron | Human Neuron |

MARVELOUS NEURONS

These diagrams are a very simple illustration of a neuron. There are many different kinds of cells in the human body and the nerve cell (neuron) is very different from all the rest, but like all body cells, it has a central body and nucleus which is the control center. It is estimated that it would require 100,000 pages of small print to contain all of the information to be found in just one neuron. Now multiply that by ten to twelve billion neurons in the nervous system! ! You don't mind if I take just a moment to stop and enjoy the marvels of our Creator's handiwork? Really? OK! You remember we mentioned the lowly earthworm with only 20 neurons? What instincts, reflexes, mobility, metabolic provisions, propagation capabilities and many other provisions it displayed all with only 20 neurons. Just think about the honey bee in flight, operating four tiny wings and coordinating its many tiny muscles enabling it to fly forward, backward, hover motionless, negotiating directly into the center of a blossom waving in the wind, communicating with other bees in some kind of meaningful language, telling them what to do and where they found the best nectar. They analyze earth's magnetic fields to tell direction, they compensate for wind velocity and direction so as never to get lost. They are keenly sensitive to sound, odors, ultraviolet light, demonstrate loyalties and adhere to the laws of the colony. They are clever architects, they accomplish their propagational secrets and much, much more and with less than a thousand neurons. All this is contained in a brain the size of a grain of salt in that little insect's head! We could consider the ant too, "thou Sluggard!" (Proverbs 6:6)

What must be the potential of the human brain with its ten or more billion neurons? We are told that on the average we use about four percent of them. What did God have in mind when He created man? Surely He didn't intend that 96% of our neurons remain idle. Have you heard that, "An idle mind is the devil's workshop?" On the other hand, have you heard, "Christ can and will, if we submit to Him, fill the chambers of the mind and every recess [100%] of our being with His Holy Spirit."[77]

Are you slowly, but surely, embracing and appreciating more and more the great wisdom of the Creator and the PROVISION He has made for our communion with Him? But we have only scratched the surface! Let us hasten on to new heights! Oh, I pray that as I write these words that you may be able to envision a little of what is discernable of the love of a Father for His children who for a little while yet must live under this tremendous cloud of earthly influences and limitations. How He longs to re-

---

lease us and gather us to Himself and nourish us until we can grow up to meet His original intent for us.

Thy People long have waited
Their absent Lord to see;
And Still in loneliness they wait
With Him to ever be.

How long Oh Lord our God,
Most holy, true and good;
Wilt Thou yet linger while You see
Our plight, our tears, our Blood?

Come Lord and wipe away
The curse, the sin, the stain,
And make this blighted world of ours
Thine own fair world again.

(Horatius Bonar, 1885)

CHAPTER ELEVEN

Consider briefly how nerve messages travel. Long before it was known that nerve messages traveled by electrical impulse, Ellen White spoke of the electrical currents of the brain. "The brain nerves which communicate with the entire system are the only medium through which heaven can communicate with man, and affect his inmost life. Whatever disturbs the circulation of the electric currents in the nervous system, lessens the strength of the vital powers, and the result is a deadening of the sensibilitities of the mind."[78]

Electric current along a nerve fiber is not like electron flow in a metal wire. Electrical power, as we are accustomed to using it, requires metal conductors; copper, aluminum, brass, etc., but not so with nerve tissue, fiberoptics notwithstanding. Nevertheless it is an electrical impulse that travels, or flows, and is a current. It is an electro-chemical arrangement. Briefly explained, there are potassium ions on the inside of the nerve fiber and saline (sodium) on the outside. A neuron at rest, therefore, has a negative charge on the inside compared to the outside, so there is a stationary electric charge that exists across the nerve wall. If the cell wall is attacked, physically, chemically, electrically, or is otherwise disturbed, it becomes more or less permeable, and depending on the intensity of the disturbance will be the degree of permeability of the neuron wall. The more intense the disturbance the more permeable the wall. The more permeable the wall the easier the sodium and potassium ions will pass through the wall. The potassium ions go through easier than the sodium ions, so the result is the polarity (the positive to negative charge) across the wall reverses. This reversal induces (influences) the ion arrangements of the neighboring wall area and it becomes more permeable so its wall polarity reverses and so on down the nerve fiber. The stronger the disturbance, the faster will be the propagation of the disturbance, varying from 2 mph to 200 mph. In the meantime after a short refractory period of about one thousandth of a second, the original point of disturbance recovers its original polarity and is ready for the next influence. So nerve messages are waves of reversing polarity, traveling along the nerve fiber. A nerve can transmit a message to its cell body, have it analyzed there and pass it on to other intended areas at the rate of about one thousand per second! *Praise God from whom all blessings FLOW!*

It is of no small point of passing interest that our Father in heaven decided to create all of our body cells, neurons included, out of light weight tissue instead of copper, and still arranged for it to carry electric currents. You might remember to thank Him tonight for that 1850 pound blessing! Imagine besides that, having to carry a lead storage battery six feet tall and four feet in circumference to furnish the power for your nervous system; another four thousand pounds. You know that could have been part of the post-Eden curse! Imagine what would have happened if after the fall, Adam had decided to jump into ye ole swimmin hole under that situation! "China, here I come!" Perish the thought and pardon the side track. At least don't let that nerve impulse spread its influence any further.

CHAPTER TWELVE

By now you are prepared for the most thrilling and applicable anatomy of all. Suppose that just now a message, an electrical impulse, is coming along a nerve fiber, maybe slowly, maybe rapidly, depending on its voltage and on the diameter of the axon fiber carrying it. As the axon winds its way through the millions of interlacing fibers of other neurons, it follows on till it reaches the end of the axon where it connects with the receptor end (the dendrite) of another neuron, or with many other dendrites. But it does not quite connect. There is a very small gap preventing a real connection. That little gap between the axon of one neuron and the dendrite of the next neuron is called the SYNAPSE. Someone has suggested that the Synapse surely is the most important single determinant entity of all of human life! As we continue I think you will agree. Let us look into the strange activities that give this tiny gap such a ponderous reputation. Another has called it "The port of every origin and the harbor of every destiny." Still another has said, "Here every thought has its birth and every act earns its judgment."

What happens when a message, sometimes called an impulse or an action potential, arrives at this gap—the Synapse? Will it jump the gap or will it be a wasted effort; a call for action that was never delivered? As you might guess, one factor in the success of the message getting across the gap would be its strength (voltage), another its speed, another would be the nature of the fluid in which the gap is immersed, and finally what kind of a welcome will it find on the other side of the gap?

Synapses (that's plural for synapse) have certain chemical characteristics that are always present in plenteous supply, but also certain electrical characteristics that are present in more or less plenteous supply depending on the previous experience of the Synapse.

Some of its experiences may have been of quite recent occurrence, maybe one hundred fiftieth of a second ago, while some of them may have occurred half a lifetime in the past. What a unique opportunity for our Creator to erect a road sign; "Guard well the avenues of the soul."[79] Yes, at the Synapse. "Gird up the loins of your mind." (1Peter 1:13) Mind? Yes, that's where you find the Synapses. Remember what we learned, "The Synapse is the most important single determinant entity of all of human life."—very, very, true.

Here the message stands and it will die in about 15 milliseconds (one seventieth of a second) if not delivered, but here a wonderful series of events are ready to take over.

The Synapse maintains a certain minimum threshold voltage, called a "bias" voltage, that prevents any and all message impulses from passing through it unless they are of a certain minimal strength. This is to prevent low level background confusion from interfering with clear reception! (I thought RCA invented that! No! It's very old! They learned it from our Father.) For example, suppose the bias voltage is 20 mv. (20 millivolts). That's 2/100 of a volt. Not much for sure, but just right. So any incoming signal must be at least 20 mv. or more to get through the Synapse. A 15 mv. message doesn't stand a chance, but you remember the little fellow can live for 15 milliseconds (1/70 second) and if another message from the same source and bearing the identical message can arrive within that time, it adds up to 2 x 15 mv. = 30 mv., and that easily overcomes the 20 mv. bias against the message, and away it goes through the gate, pardon me, gap, pardon me, Synapse. Why do I capitalize Synapse all the time? I just figure it's that important, every bit that important, besides my Father says it's every bit that important. "In **all** thy **ways** acknowledge Him and He shall direct thy <u>PATHS</u>." (Proverbs 3:6) As I was about to say, this quick succession of the arrival of impulses is called <u>Repetive Summation</u>. Fancy name and I wouldn't mention it, except that there is another one called <u>Tempo-ral Summation</u>, that says, if two messages from **different** sources, but bearing the same credentials and arriving within 15 milliseconds of each other, they can combine their voltages and gain access. Now God intended it for good, but as usual the devil knows about it, but praise the Lord there is another surprise just waiting to spring up.

Are you with me? The next interesting step? "<u>Very</u>" interesting!

There are two other biases (voltages) that a Synapse may generate, "Oh No! Not more Physics and Chemistry and Math., I can't enjoy the forest for all the trees in the way. Hang on! Trees are what the forest is made of, and the forest is about to appear in all of its beauty.

As I was saying, there are two other bias voltages that a Synapse may bring into play if it so chooses, or more exactly, if it has been <u>taught</u> to bring them into play; taught by previous experiences. These two other biases have highly suggestive names; <u>Facilitory</u> and <u>Inhibitory</u> biases or voltages, and they impress themselves on the incoming impulses in the same manner as the bias that we previously mentioned. It is simply a matter of total-ling up the pluses and minuses to see who wins. The Fa-cilitory bias helps open the gate of the Synapse and the Inhibitory bias tries to keep the Synapse closed, and it depends upon the sum of all the bias influences whether the message will be received or rejected. These Facilitory and Inhibitory influences are programmed by the higher decision areas of the CNS. In time the Synapse will begin to act independently on its own initiative; "habituated" to act as it has been influenced on previous occasions from the higher centers, such that habits are formed to receive or reject all future influences based on its past instructions. Eventually the Synapse becomes practical-ly a perfect conductor or a perfect insulator as it learns to recognize the nature of the incoming message and responds according to the WILL of the higher centers without having to pause to consult the higher centers. "Likewise reckon ye also yourselves to be dead indeed to

sin, but alive unto God through Jesus Christ our Lord."
(Romans 6:11) and "Whosoever is born of God doth not
commit sin for his seed remaineth in him and he cannot sin!"—wholly (holy) <u>Facilitated</u>! Thus a habit, well
formed, becomes a character as far as that particular
small microscopic increment of the nervous system is
concerned, and the higher centers can march on to still
higher considerations. How high, Father?

I'm pressing on the upward way,
  New heights I'm gaining every day;
   Still praying as i onward bound,
    Lord plant my feet on higher ground

   My heart has no desire to stay,
    Where doubts arise and fears dismay;
     Though some may dwell where these abound,
    My prayer, my aim is higher ground

    I want to live above the world,
     Though Satan's darts at me are hurled;
      For faith has caught the joyful sound,
      The song of saints, on higher ground
             —Johnson Oatman, Jr. 1896

    Let's play games! No, let's not play games! Life is not
a game, it's a predetermined destiny!—"for whatsoever a
man soweth, that shall he also reap." (Galatians 6:7) Predetermined? Yes. Let's suppose a 75 mv. (between meals)
hunger impulse comes temptingly up to a Synapse and
meets the 20 mv. opposing bias. No problem it thinks,
but a 60mv. <u>Inhibitory</u> bias joins the 20 mv. standard bias
which all adds up to 80 mv. and the 75 mv. impulse is
repulsed. Barely repulsed, I might add. It is always true,
the stronger the preparation, the more certain the victory.
That 60 mv. Inhibitory bias may have been accumulated
there over the past few days or it may have been there
since childhood, but it must be reviewed, put in remem-
brance and if necessary established under persecution,
for if left unattended it will fade.

Again an interesting situation: A weak 15 mv. impulse to eat between meals. The standard 20 mv. bias can easily oppose the decision, but that person is a highly nervous individual which may add 10 mv. of nervousness to the temptation, which added to the weak 15 mv. temptation, makes a total of 25 mv., overcomes the 20 mv. bias, the person grabs the candy bar and adds to the undesirable programming of the Synapse for the next candy bar. "0 wretched man that I am! Who shall save me...? I thank God, through Jesus Christ our Lord." (Romans 7: 24,25) He does not approve of hasty and nervous decisions.

Among other influences, caffeine (coffee), xanthine (tea), amphetamines, and alkalines, stimulate (Facilitate) the passage of nerve impulses, while hypnotics, sedatives, narcotics, anesthesia and acidosis, depress (Inhibitory bias) the passage of nerve impulses. The "road sign" here should read, "Avoid stimulants and avoid depressants, tranquilizers and soporifics and above all remember what happened the last time you stood at this fork in the road."

CHAPTER THIRTEEN

You have heard a person speak who stutters or stammers? Fortunately the <u>healthy</u> Synapse under <u>normal</u> conditions becomes fatigued in about 1/1000 of a second. Nerve fibers do not fatigue, but the Synapse does very rapidly and is ready for the next impulse. Yes, the Synapse fatigues rapidly, otherwise if it didn't and you started to say "Abraham," you would get to "A" and be stuck at "AAAAA"! Mississippi would be more comfortable, MM-MMM—. If you looked at a picture of an iceberg, your vision would be locked in on it; frozen if you please. You would see nothing else, even though you turned your eyes to look at a bonfire! If you reached up to catch an incoming baseball, that would be the end of the game I suppose! So fortunately, in most cases the Synapse is quick to make up its "mind" and release the impulse.

Discussing the characteristics of the Synapse—yes, Synapses do have character; where else is your character? Your eternal destiny depends on the sum-total of all your totally <u>Facilitated</u> and all of your totally <u>Inhibited</u> Synapses! This is your character, the sum of all their characters! Oh yes, we started to discuss the characteristics of the Synapse. We have already determined (mathematically) that the stronger the message, the greater the probability of its getting through the Synapse. Also the more frequent the review, the more automatic and perfect the habituated response.

If I say, "Red, white and _____, "you automatically say, " Blue."

If I say, "Matthew, Mark, Luke and _____," you automatically say, John."

If I say, "Roses are red _____," you automatically say, "Violets are blue."

Why? Because you have done it so many times before. Each passing of the message leaves its foot print.

You have tramped a "rut" through the Synapse. A totally Facilitated Synapse. So completely facilitated that it is quite certain that you will never forget those three phrases. Which reminds me of another phrase that applies to the Synapse; "Practice makes perfect." This brings us to a most profound observation. If practice makes perfect, then the very first act of that practice must have at least an infinitesimal effect. There is a law of our nature, written in our Synapses, that decrees that we can never be exactly the same after facing a situation that requires a decision. We will either be more certain that we made the right decision or we will be less certain. We will never be the same after facing temptation. We will either gain a victory and be stronger for the next assault or we will be weaker for the next one we face. "Those who indulge known sin will be more readily overcome the second time. The first transgression opens the door to the tempter and he gradually breaks down all resistance and takes full possession of the citadel of the soul."[80]

Reason, judgment and conscience are the result of previous neurological experiences and that comes with time and maturity, but reason, judgement and conscience can only recommend to us. The WILL determines what shall be done. "...It is the governing power in the nature of men."[81]

The longer that reason, judgment, conscious and the WILL remain fixed in a given pattern, the more fixed and permanently established will be the Character. **Character** is that fixed attitude and response of a person that results from the repeated and habitual application of the WILL. This is what caused Martin Luther to say, "I cannot, I **will** not retract. It is unsafe for a Christian to speak against his conscience. Here I stand. I can do no other. May God help me. Amen."

If we can say that the **REAL YOU** and the **REAL ME** are the result of all of our billions of Synaptic thought and action patterns, our memory patterns, our habit pat-

---

80   *Conflict and Courage,* 119
81   *Education,* 289

terns, our moral standards, our reasoning patterns, our judgmental methods, our conscience and our WILL, then we should be able to understand in a new light such sentences, quotes, phrases or other reminders that we have heard so often before, such as: "I delight to do Thy will, Oh my God. Yea, Thy law is [programmed] within my heart [CNS]." "Thy Word have I hidden [programmed] in my heart [CNS], that I might not sin against Thee." (Psalms 119:11)

God provides power for victory day by day; Facilitative and Inhibitory bias. This is not a psychological mind trip, but a living electro-chemical experience at the Synapse, dependent upon a continuous relationship with a Person. If we take control by persistently acting against anyone's will, our relationship with that person will soon end. If we are "born again," we will not desire to "Interpose our perverse will and thus frustrate His grace."[82] We will not want to break that close relationship with Christ, because He is in control of all our Synaptic decision patterns. "His seed [His decisions] remaineth in us and we <u>cannot</u> sin, for we are born of God" (pronouns altered) (1John 3:9), because we know if we do, that relation will be broken and we would rather die than to have that happen. We talk about assigning our will to God. It is a yearning that only right shall prevail, only right shall be recognized for passage through any Synapse. Is our Father concerned for our success in setting up this structure of our CNS? "Tenderly He watches over you, every <u>Facilitation</u>, every <u>Inhibition</u> of the way." "Christ's love vitalizes the nerves." "Let every nerve <u>respond</u> to the expression of God's love."[83] "God's laws are written upon every nerve." "The love of God must sweep through the chambers of the mind."[84] "Often there will come to us a sweet, joyful sense of the presence of Jesus." "Christ can and will, if we submit to Him fill the chambers of the mind and every recess of the being with His Holy

---

82   *Mount of Blessings*, 76
83   *Testimonies*, Volume 4, 581
84   *God's Amazing Grace*, 206

Spirit."[85] "It is the privilege of every Christian to experience the deep movings of the holy Spirit upon the heart
[mind]."[86] "In all thy [nerve ways] acknowledge Him and
He shall direct thy [nerve paths]." (Proverbs 3:6) "Hedge
up the <u>way</u> with, it is written."[87]

Oh, there must be "a voice crying in the wilderness
[of our 10 billion neurons], <u>program</u> ye the nerve-way
of the Lord, 'make straight in the desert [of our mind] a
highway for our God." (Isaiah 39:3)

Henceforth let every thing we read of God's Word,
hold a more meaningful and appreciative application to
our anatomy,—*The Anatomy Of A Christian*. Let every
phrase of the words of inspiration enter into our weaving
of personally and permanently facilitated nervous pathways through our Synapses.

85   *Our High Calling*, 219
86   *God's Amazing Grace*, 318
87   Ibid., 262

CHAPTER FOURTEEN

All habits, good or bad, require time to become firmly "fixed." The Synapse requires time to become strongly <u>facilitated</u> or firmly <u>inhibited</u>.

Good habits require more time.

Bad habits require less time.

<u>Why the difference</u>?

<u>BECAUSE</u>

God gave you a WILL
AND
God respects your WILL

God gave you a WILL
BUT
Satan <u>doesn't</u> respect your WILL

GOD
Always "plays fair"
Always "out in the open"
Always "above board"
Never rushes you
Never forces you

SATAN
"Plays dirty tricks"
Pushes in on you
Always behind your back
Sneaks in the "back door"
Catches you "off guard"
Tries to embarrass you
Says, "Just this once"

Yes, God plays fair. He knocks on the door. We are the one who opens the door, otherwise He stays outside. He never forces His way inside. "Behold I stand at the door and knock. If any man hear My voice and open the door, I will come in..." (Revelation 3:20)

Satan never knocks on the door, never announces himself. He sneaks in the back door and waits until our guard is down a little; maybe just a little spiritually asleep, if for only a moment.

How often have we repeated, "Good habits require time and repetition?" "It takes time to transform the human to the divine, or to degrade those formed in the image of God to the brute and Satanic. By beholding we become changed... Character does not come by chance... It is the repetition of the act that caused it to become a habit and mold the character for good or for evil. Right characters are formed only by persevering, untiring effort."[91]

Sow a thought	Reap an act.
Sow an act	Reap a habit.
Sow a habit	Reap a character.
Sow a character	Reap a destiny.

Always keep in mind the transforming processes that are continually adjusting themselves every second in your delicate nervous system. "Bring every thought into captivity to the obedience of Christ." (2 Corinthians, 10:5) Invite Jesus to walk with you as He develops in you His choices for you. "Christ will abide in you. He will put His hand to the work of creating you anew."[92] Thrill to that thought for a moment and in your imagination try to hear the turmoil among the Synapses, being "born again!" Is the Holy Spirit creating you anew this very minute? There is a great work to be done. There is a quick work to be done. How can it be quick, you ask, with ten to twelve billion Synapses to be readjusted? That is a hopeless task, you say, an endless job? Take heart dear friend. Gaining the victory over appetite alone will account for the correction of about one billion neurons! "The mind in which Jesus makes His abode will be quickly purified, guided and ruled by the Holy Spirit."[93]

91   *God's Amazing Grace*, 224
92   *In Heavenly Places*, 64
93   *God's Amazing Grace*, 206

Oh the joy that transcends earthliness and the peace that surpasses worldly understanding. Let the language of the soul be, "Lo God is at work here."

We will pause a moment to take note of a few promises that in the context of our new understanding of the activities transpiring in our nervous system, we will enjoy a deeper understanding of the **reality** of God's plan for sanctifying our CNS!

1. "Man has the power to control and regulate the working of the mind and to give **direction to the current** of his thoughts...The mind is so constructed that it must be occupied by either **good** or **evil** therefore we must **stay** our mind on God."[94]

2. "In order to understand this matter aright, we must remember that our hearts [minds] are **naturally** depraved and we are unable of ourselves to pursue a right course...without the Holy Spirit we have no power against Satan."[95]

3. "Men with Spiritual nerves are needed to resist Satan's artifices."[96]

4. "If we consent, He will so identify Himself with our **thoughts** and so blend our hearts and **minds** into conformity with His will, that when obeying Him we shall be but carrying out our own **impulses**."[97]

5. The **new birth** is brought about by the effectual working of the Holy Spirit on the **mind**."[98]

---

94   Ibid., 258
95   *Counsels to Parents, Teachers and Students*, 544
96   *Testimonies*, Volume 4, 155
97   *Desire of Ages*, 688
98   *God's Amazing Grace*, 22

6. "Let the language of the heart be, 'Lo God is here. The Lord is in His holy temple, let all the earth keep silence before Him.'"[99]

7. "Many have made a habit of pursuing a course of sin and their minds **harden** [totally facilitated to evil] under Satan's influence, but when they place their minds against the temptations of Satan, their minds are made **clear** [Synapse opened] and their conscience made sensitive....and sin then appears as it is—exceedingly sinful...Those who walk in wisdom's way are, even in tribulation, exceeding joyful, for He whom their soul loveth, **walks invisible** beside them. At each upward step they discern more distinctly the touch of His hand, and hear His voice say, 'This is the **way**, walk ye in it.'"[100]

8. Circumcise [purify] the foreskin [forebrain] of your heart [mind] and be no more stiff necked [basal ganglia controlled.] (Deuteronomy 10:16)

9. "It is our privilege to have a living, abiding Saviour **implanted within us**...an indwelling Saviour."[101]

10. "Every Christian must stand on guard, continually watching every **avenue** of the soul...Let him remember, Christ must **abide within** him."[102]

11. "The Holy Spirit is to be continually with the believer. We have need to more carefully consider the fact the Comforter is to abide **in** us."[103]

---

99   Ibid., 202
100   Ibid., 264
101   Ibid., 119
102   *Testimonies*, Volume 5, 47, 48
103   *Faith I Live By*, 57

CHAPTER FIFTEEN

We have learned that it requires time to form habits; time for frequent review; for re-thinking; for re-examining; for re-adjusting; for re-affirming.

FORMING GOOD HABITS: Good habits are formed by frequently conditioning the Synapse to recognize good incoming impulses, such that they do not excite **inhibitory** biases (excuses) against their passage. It is a settling into the truth, both intellectually and spiritually; a settling into unchanging **molds** such that we cannot be moved.

"To dwell upon the beauty, goodness, mercy and love of Jesus is strengthening to the mental powers and while the mind is kept **training** to do the works of Christ and to be obedient children, you will habitually inquire, 'Is this the **way** [nerve pathway] of the Lord; would Jesus be pleased this way?"[104] [Have I properly programmed my Reticular System this **way**?]

"All the **way** up the steep road to eternal life...He Whom their soul loveth **walks invisible** beside them."[105]

"Good habits are best formed as we submit to the moment by moment leading of the Holy Spirit. This means perfect love, perfect obedience, perfect conformity to the will of God."[106]

OVERCOMING BAD HABITS: Again it requires time to overcome a bad habit; time to constantly deny their passage through the Synapse; time to program the Reticulum such that it will respond properly and automatically. (Remember the Reticulum is the center which is trained by the higher centers to automatically respond in the manner that is has previously been taught to respond,

---

104   *God's Amazing Grace*, 264
105   Ibid., 264
106   *Acts of the Apostles*, 565

without the higher centers having to even be conscious of a decision having been made and acted upon.) Do not review bad habits, but deny them. Sometimes **trying** to deny them only brings them into sharper focus; a stronger and tempting memory of them; so in such cases substitution of a good act to compete with the bad act is the only way out. "Be not overcome with evil but overcome evil with good." (Romans 12:21) "Guard well the **avenues** of the soul."[107]

"Every act of self denial for His sake, every trial well endured, every victory gained over temptation, is a step in the march to the glory of final victory."[108]

GOOD MEMORY: A good memory is the result of Synapses that are so completely conditioned that there is no **inhibitory** bias, and on the other hand such a strong **facilitory** charge that when an impulse arrives even related neighboring Synapses "fire across," coming to the rescue and encourage by creating parallel pathways for identical impulses. The mere suggestion of an event sets off a whole host of related memories and responses which are rapidly passed through their respective Synapses and the whole original setting with all of the fine details passes in review before the memory screen of the brain. An example may be the overwhelming denial of a temptation to a sinful act or perhaps a strong supportive response to a proper appeal.

Under the heading of a good memory is a phenomenon that might be called the "carry on" memory. It is not unusual to observe this "carry on" memory in action. You readily recall that certain acquaintance who will "pick up" on a word that you might mention and "carry on" a conversation ad infinitum that your word stimulated. The flow of words rambles from one subject to another as memory reviews itself from one pathway to another. An extreme example of the "carry on" memory is the case of a person who calls with nothing more important than to

---

107   *Patriarchs*, 460
108   *God's Amazing Grace*, 264

say, "Hello," but who rambles on for an hour or more. The party on the receiving end of the line lays his phone down and allows the memory review to coast on and on. Every five or ten minutes he picks up the phone and says, "uh-huh" then lays the phone down again and continues his work. Finally he starts dialing at random and the "carry on" caller says, "Oh, someone must be trying to call you, I'd better let you go." Unusual? Not at all!

A good memory is one of the greatest assets an individual can possess. It must be encouraged. Memory is best supported by relating new inputs with older, easily recalled memories. There are many methods of developing "recall." Most people invent their own methods, but the primary and best method is a permanently **facilitated** Synapse.

FORGETTING: The Synapse, we have learned, is the point of communication between neurons, and if at this interchange an event is "recorded" and frequently reviewed, the memory of it will be prolonged. On the contrary, if the event is not reviewed and not "brought to mind" for a time, the record will begin to fade and will eventually be entirely forgotten. The more forcefully the original event was impressed, the longer the imprint will be retained, but a mere "passing fancy" will soon be lost.

Frequent recall defeats the fading memory (the forgetting phenomenon). So, "Let us keep the treasure house of the mind filled with, 'It is written.' Hang in memory's hall the precious words of Christ."[109]

We have all experienced the situation of trying to recall a name, but can't quite pull it out of the maze, and the harder one tries the more frustrated one becomes. Frustration is a nervous **inhibitory** bias and is the basis for the inability to recall. If one stops trying to recall and thinks of something else for a moment, suddenly the name flashes through the unguarded, relaxed Synapse.

---

109   *Ministry of Healing*, 215

This previous frustration situation is often referred to as "jamming" of the Synapse.

The best method of erasing (purposely forgetting) a bad memory is to compete with good ones. One **cannot try** to forget. That only reinforces memory. God did not install a primary "forgetter" in our CNS. One can build up **inhibitory** bias voltages to evil, but one cannot forget by intention; only by competition. As we have said, "Be not overcome with evil but overcome evil with good." (Revelation 12:21)

CHAPTER SIXTEEN

At this stage in our study the question again surfaces: Can we explain the working of the Holy Spirit on the Mind? The straight, firm and never changing answer is: No, not at all." The best and nearest that we can ever do, and that we are invited to do is, to **experience** it and to do that which we have been doing:

1.) **Study the inspired Word** for the **evidences** that God does desire to **indwell** us and commune with us.

2.) **Study our Person** for evidence of a **PROVISION** for the indwelling of His Holy Spirit.

Following through on these two approaches:

1.) In our **study of the Word**, we have found that God **does** strongly indicate His desire to indwell and communicate with us.

2.) In the **study of our Person,** we have learned that there is a **PROVISION**, a marvelous and delicate provision for the introduction and transport of messages to every cell of the body.

We have learned that the nervous system has two general divisions. One division is entirely automatic and which is called the **Autonomic Nervous System** or **Involuntary Nervous System**, while the other division of the CNS is **not** automatic and is called the **Voluntary Nervous System** and which calls for a "director."

It seems that in the creation process of the human nervous system, God took care of every minute detail in it except for one thing. Did God forget something? No indeed! This is the place where He again chose to display

His great love and wisdom. He took care of everything, but left one little spot that requires a director. The director, He deliberately left for us to choose. Then, right there at that very spot and in plain sight, He left a "road sign." On the sign He wrote His carefully worded and inspired instructions, which says, "Study to show thyself approved unto [Me], a workman that needeth not to be ashamed, rightly dividing the Word of Truth." (2 Timothy, 2:15), and signed it, "For you My Child, from your Father."

> *Behold what manner of love*
> *The Father hath bestowed upon us,*
> *That we should be called*
> *"THE SONS OF GOD!"*
> (1 John, 3:1)

CHAPTER SEVENTEEN

In summary: Our study of the nervous system of the human body reveals a widespread system of delicate communication capabilities that provide checks and balances, covering the needs of every cell of the body except those billions of "gaps" in the system. Those gaps, the Synapses, reserve the ability to conduct or not to conduct electro-chemical impulses across themselves. Their decision whether to convey or not to convey these messages seems to rest on a very delicate decision based on "**NEED.**" The **simple needs** for satisfaction and promotion of the basic life processes are automatic and are apparently "built into" the system and perpetuates itself. This self-perpetuating provision is, as we have learned, is the "Autonomics;" the involuntary nervous system.

The **higher** levels of decision and control that require a **director** outside of itself, is left to the constituency of that portion of the system that is not automatic, the "voluntary nervous system." The constituency has the property of being aware of (conscious of) its surroundings and immediate needs. It is unable of itself to control its long term needs, ie, its eventual destiny. It may recognize that fact or it may not recognize it. The Creator knows what is best for its control, but does not force His directorship on the voluntary portion of the nervous system. Unfortunately there is a competitor for the Creator's control of the system, and the competitor's desire is to eventually destroy the system, but intends to deceive the system of that fact. The Creator or the deceiver, either one is stronger in ability to control the system than the system itself is to control itself, so one or the other of the two competitors is automatically the controller.

Fortunately, the Creator is the stronger of the two competitors, but He is also the wiser and has arranged that the system **can** freely choose (not **must** choose) which director it will have to rule over it. The Creator has said that those who desire His directorship must declare their decision to Him. He will not force Himself on them. Failure to choose the Creator results in the competitor taking charge by default, and he will do so without a request, for he is an unfair actor. The Creator asks each, "Choose ye this day whom ye will serve." (Joshua, 24:15)

"Man has the power to regulate and control the working of the mind and to **give direction** to the **current** of his thoughts, but this requires more effort than we can make in our own strength. The mind is so constituted that it must be occupied with either good or evil, therefore, we must stay our mind on God. "[110] This reminds us of the sage saying: "An idle mind is the devil's workshop."

"In order to understand the matter aright, we must remember that our hearts [minds] are naturally depraved and we are unable of ourselves to pursue a right course. It is only the grace of God combined with the utmost earnest effort on our part that we can gain the victory. Without the Holy Spirit with us, we have no power against Satan."[111]

The Synapses of the "voluntary" portion of the nervous system are controlled either by the Creator or by His competitor, the one or the other; entirely the One or the other; entirely the One or the other. Most of the world's nervous systems operate by default. They have never **chosen**, so the competitor has taken control.

We have learned that the important decisions of the WILL are made in the FORE-BRAIN; that reserved and sacred temple of the Holy Ghost. Let us not consider ourselves as an abandoned nervous system floating around until we run out of energy. We were created by a loving, caring God and intended by Him to exist for eternity, and destined to return with Him to our home of origin if we submit and assign ourselves and every living, acting cell in our body to His tender oversight and control. "We are bound to give thanks always to God for you, brethren

---

110   *God's Amazing Grace*, 258
111   *Counsels to Parents, Teachers and Students*, 544

beloved of the Lord, because God hath from the beginning chosen you to salvation through sanctification of the Spirit and belief of the truth." (2 Thessalonians 2:13)

Truly each and every Synapse is a very special gift of our Creator, each one intended and invited to **yield** to its Creator's Will. It is our privilege to assign it and to "will" it to His care.

Henceforth, read with new insight, the comments and invitations from the inspired words of the prophets. Sing with new understanding the old songs that welled up to overflowing from the hearts of poets, musicians and historians.

Live out thy life within me, O Jesus, King of kings!
Be thou Thy-self the answer to all my questionings;
Live out Thy life within me, in all things have Thy way!
I, the transparent medium Thy glory to display.

The temple has been yielded, and purified of sin;
Let Thy Shekinah glory, now shine forth from within,
And all the earth keep silence, the body henc-forth be
Thy silent gentle servant, moved only by Thee.

It's member every moment, held subject to Thy call,
Ready to have Thee use them, or not be used at all;
Held without restless longing, or strain, or stress or fret,
Or chafing at Thy dealings, or thoughts of vain regret.

But restful, calm and pliant, from bend and bias free,
A-waiting Thy decision, when Thou hast need of me.
Live out Thy life within me, O Jesus King of kings!
Be Thou the glorious answer to all my questionings.

(Samuel Wesley, 1864)

We'd love to have you download our catalog of titles we publish at:

www.TEACHServices.com

or write or email us your thoughts, reactions, or criticism about this or any other book we publish at:

TEACH Services, Inc.
254 Donovan Road
Brushton, NY 12916

info@TEACHServices.com

or you may call us at:

518/358-3494